T0381050

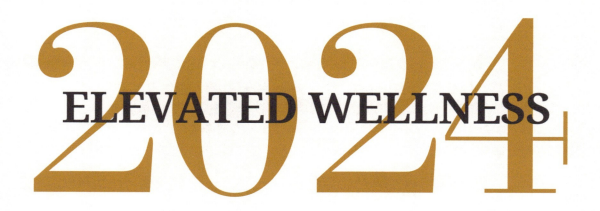

2024
ELEVATED WELLNESS

A MINDFULNESS & COGNITIVE BEHAVIORAL THERAPY WEEKLY PLANNER

Created by Jasmin James, LPC, LCDC

Introduction to the
Elevated Wellness Weekly Planner

This Mindfulness and Cognitive Behavioral Therapy (CBT) weekly planner was thoughtfully tailored for those desiring to elevate and improve their wellness in various aspects. This planner is for the person in pursuit of becoming the better version of themselves. This is where you start. This is for you!

This weekly planner is beneficial to a wide range of individuals, including but not limited to, the overthinker, the perfectionist, the people pleaser, the overachiever, the procrastinator, the indecisive, and the impulsive.
This weekly planner is for you! This is not a substitute for psychotherapy but an additive tool on your wellness journey. Let's optimize your time and get your life back!

- Mindfulness is an awareness of your internal state, emotions, thoughts, and surroundings.
- Cognitive Behavioral Therapy helps you understand the connection between your thoughts and your actions. CBT also aids in unlearning negative thoughts to decrease negative behaviors. Learning healthier thinking patterns leads to healthier habits.
- Wellness is the act of practicing healthy habits on a daily basis to attain better physical and mental health outcomes

This weekly planner was curated to help people organize their lives, develop healthy habits, and increase self-awareness. You don't need to be a mental health or wellness expert to utilize this planner. If you are ready to take your time, mind, and body back from the chaos to live more in the ease and flow of life, this weekly planner is for you.

The contents of this planner have helped me feel better about myself inside and out. My confidence has increased, I have developed and sustained a healthier mindset which led to healthier habits, and healthy relationships. Thank you for choosing to Elevate Your Wellness with me!
-
Jasmin James, LPC, LCDC

Elevated Wellness Weekly Planner

Web Resources

WWW.PSYCHOLOGYTODAY.COM
HTTPS://OPENPATHCOLLECTIVE.ORG/
HTTPS://WWW.BETTERHELP.COM/THERAPISTS/
HTTPS://WWW.TALKSPACE.COM/
HTTPS://HEADWAY.CO/
HTTPS://THERAPYFORBLACKMEN.ORG/
HTTPS://THERAPYFORBLACKGIRLS.COM/

Phone Resources

National Suicide Hotline- 1-800-273-8255
National Domestic Violence Hotline- 1-800-799-7233
National Sexual Assault Hotline- 1-800-656-4673
National Crisis Line- 988
National Crisis Text line- Text HOME to 741741 (United States)

I WOULD LIKE TO GIVE A **SINCERE** AND **HUGE THANK YOU** TO THE INCREDIBLE ARTIST LEO, ALSO KNOW AS, SOLEOADO.
LEO GRACIOUSLY GRANTED PERMISSION FOR THEIR WORK TO BE SHOWCASED IN THIS WEEKLY PLANNER.
THEIR WORK SPEAKS TO THE HEART OF THIS PROJECT, WHICH IS WELLNESS, LOVE, LIFE, STRENGTH, JOY, FREEDOM, AND GREATNESS!
YOU CAN FIND MORE OF LEO'S WORK ON INSTAGRAM AND FACEBOOK FOR PURCHASE AND SUPPORT.

THANK YOU AGAIN, LEO FOR SHARING YOUR TALENT AND SPIRIT WITH ME AND MORE IMPORTANTLY THE WORLD!

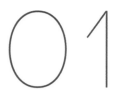

01

JANUARY
2024

SUNDAY	MONDAY	TUESDAY	WEDNESDAY	THURSDAY	FRIDAY	SATURDAY
	1	2	3	4	5	6
7	8	9	10	11	12	13
14	15	16	17	18	19	20
21	22	23	24	25	26	27
28	29	30	31			

HABITS TO START

- _____
- _____
- _____

HABITS TO STOP

- _____
- _____
- _____

SELF-CARE ACTIVITIES

- _____
- _____
- _____

DON'T FORGET

WEEKLY PLAN

THIS WEEKS PRIORITIES/GOALS

○ _____
○ _____
○ _____
○ _____
○ _____
○ _____
○ _____
○ _____

APPOINTMENTS

○ _____
○ _____
○ _____

REMINDERS

○ _____
○ _____
○ _____

THIS WEEKS
AFFIRMATION/MOTIVATION

_____

_____

_____

MONDAY   DATE: _____

_____

_____

TUESDAY   DATE: _____

_____

_____

WEDNESDAY   DATE: _____

_____

_____

THURSDAY   DATE: _____

_____

_____

FRIDAY   DATE: _____

_____

_____

SATURDAY   DATE: _____

_____

_____

SUNDAY   DATE: _____

_____

_____

WEEKLY PLAN

THIS WEEKS PRIORITIES/GOALS

○ _____
○ _____
○ _____
○ _____
○ _____
○ _____
○ _____
○ _____

APPOINTMENTS

○ _____
○ _____
○ _____

REMINDERS

○ _____
○ _____
○ _____

THIS WEEKS
AFFIRMATION/MOTIVATION
_____

_____

_____

_____

MONDAY   DATE: _____

_____

_____

TUESDAY   DATE: _____

_____

_____

WEDNESDAY   DATE: _____

_____

_____

THURSDAY   DATE: _____

_____

_____

FRIDAY   DATE: _____

_____

_____

SATURDAY   DATE: _____

_____

_____

SUNDAY   DATE: _____

_____

_____

WEEKLY PLAN

THIS WEEKS PRIORITIES/GOALS

○ _____
○ _____
○ _____
○ _____
○ _____
○ _____
○ _____
○ _____

APPOINTMENTS

○ _____
○ _____
○ _____

REMINDERS

○ _____
○ _____
○ _____

THIS WEEKS
AFFIRMATION/MOTIVATION

_____

_____

_____

MONDAY   DATE: _____

_____

_____

TUESDAY   DATE: _____

_____

_____

WEDNESDAY   DATE: _____

_____

_____

THURSDAY   DATE: _____

_____

_____

FRIDAY   DATE: _____

_____

_____

SATURDAY   DATE: _____

_____

_____

SUNDAY   DATE: _____

_____

_____

WEEKLY PLAN

THIS WEEKS PRIORITIES/GOALS

○ _____

○ _____

○ _____

○ _____

○ _____

○ _____

○ _____

○ _____

APPOINTMENTS

○ _____

○ _____

○ _____

REMINDERS

○ _____

○ _____

○ _____

THIS WEEKS
AFFIRMATION/MOTIVATION

_____

_____

_____

_____

MONDAY   DATE: _____

_____

_____

TUESDAY   DATE: _____

_____

_____

WEDNESDAY   DATE: _____

_____

_____

THURSDAY   DATE: _____

_____

_____

FRIDAY   DATE: _____

_____

_____

SATURDAY   DATE: _____

_____

_____

SUNDAY   DATE: _____

_____

_____

WEEKLY PLAN

THIS WEEKS PRIORITIES/GOALS

- ○ _____
- ○ _____
- ○ _____
- ○ _____
- ○ _____
- ○ _____
- ○ _____
- ○ _____

APPOINTMENTS

- ○ _____
- ○ _____
- ○ _____

REMINDERS

- ○ _____
- ○ _____
- ○ _____

THIS WEEKS
AFFIRMATION/MOTIVATION

_____

_____

_____

_____

MONDAY   DATE: _____

_____

_____

TUESDAY   DATE: _____

_____

_____

WEDNESDAY   DATE: _____

_____

_____

THURSDAY   DATE: _____

_____

_____

FRIDAY   DATE: _____

_____

_____

SATURDAY   DATE: _____

_____

_____

SUNDAY   DATE: _____

_____

_____

JOURNAL ENTRY

WHAT IS YOUR FIRST THOUGHT WHEN YOU WAKE UP? HOW WOULD YOU LIKE TO CHANGE AND/OR IMPROVE IT?

Monthly BUDGET PLANNER

📅 MONTH (CIRCLE)

JAN	FEB	MAR	APR	MAY	JUN	JUL	AUG	SEP	OCT	NOV	DEC

☰ INCOME

DATE	DESCRIPTION	AMOUNT
	TOTAL:	

🛍 EXPENSES

DATE	DESCRIPTION	AMOUNT
	TOTAL:	

⭐ SUMMARY

TOTAL INCOME	TOTAL EXPENSES	TOTAL SAVINGS

✏ NOTES

_____

_____

_____

_____

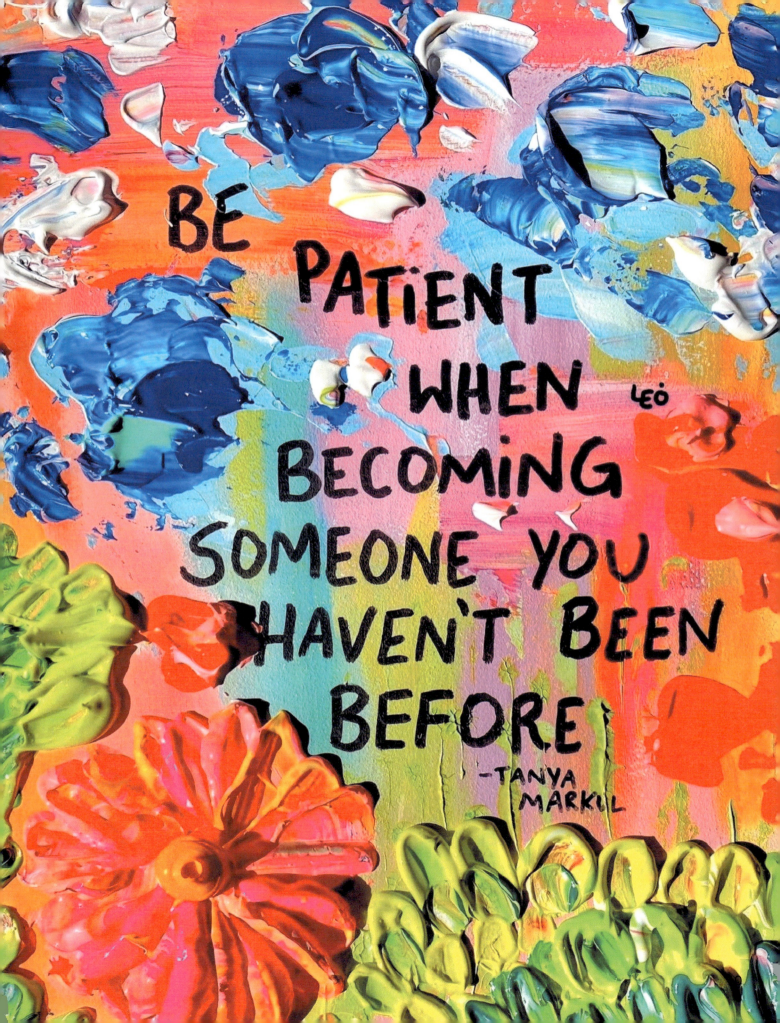

BE PATIENT WHEN BECOMING SOMEONE YOU HAVEN'T BEEN BEFORE

—TANYA MARKUL

02

SUNDAY	MONDAY	TUESDAY	WEDNESDAY	THURSDAY	FRIDAY	SATURDAY
				1	2	3
4	5	6	7	8	9	10
11	12	13	14	15	16	17
18	19	20	21	22	23	24
25	26	27	28	29		

HABITS TO START

- _____
- _____
- _____

HABITS TO STOP

- _____
- _____
- _____

SELF-CARE ACTIVITIES

- _____
- _____
- _____

DON'T FORGET

WEEKLY PLAN

THIS WEEKS PRIORITIES/GOALS

○ _____
○ _____
○ _____
○ _____
○ _____
○ _____
○ _____
○ _____

APPOINTMENTS

○ _____
○ _____
○ _____

REMINDERS

○ _____
○ _____
○ _____

THIS WEEKS
AFFIRMATION/MOTIVATION

_____

_____

_____

MONDAY   DATE: _____

_____

_____

TUESDAY   DATE: _____

_____

_____

WEDNESDAY   DATE: _____

_____

_____

THURSDAY   DATE: _____

_____

_____

FRIDAY   DATE: _____

_____

_____

SATURDAY   DATE: _____

_____

_____

SUNDAY   DATE: _____

_____

_____

WEEKLY PLAN

THIS WEEKS PRIORITIES/GOALS

○ _____
○ _____
○ _____
○ _____
○ _____
○ _____
○ _____
○ _____

APPOINTMENTS

○ _____
○ _____
○ _____

REMINDERS

○ _____
○ _____
○ _____

THIS WEEKS
AFFIRMATION/MOTIVATION
_____

_____

_____

_____

MONDAY   DATE: _____

_____

_____

TUESDAY   DATE: _____

_____

_____

WEDNESDAY   DATE: _____

_____

_____

THURSDAY   DATE: _____

_____

_____

FRIDAY   DATE: _____

_____

_____

SATURDAY   DATE: _____

_____

_____

SUNDAY   DATE: _____

_____

_____

WEEKLY PLAN

THIS WEEKS PRIORITIES/GOALS

○ _____
○ _____
○ _____
○ _____
○ _____
○ _____
○ _____
○ _____

APPOINTMENTS

○ _____
○ _____
○ _____

REMINDERS

○ _____
○ _____
○ _____

THIS WEEKS
AFFIRMATION/MOTIVATION

_____

_____

_____

MONDAY   DATE: _____

_____

_____

TUESDAY   DATE: _____

_____

_____

WEDNESDAY DATE: _____

_____

_____

THURSDAY   DATE: _____

_____

_____

FRIDAY   DATE: _____

_____

_____

SATURDAY   DATE: _____

_____

_____

SUNDAY   DATE: _____

_____

_____

WEEKLY PLAN

THIS WEEKS PRIORITIES/GOALS

○ _____
○ _____
○ _____
○ _____
○ _____
○ _____
○ _____
○ _____

APPOINTMENTS

○ _____
○ _____
○ _____

REMINDERS

○ _____
○ _____
○ _____

THIS WEEKS
AFFIRMATION/MOTIVATION
_____

_____

_____

MONDAY   DATE: _____
_____
_____

TUESDAY   DATE: _____
_____
_____

WEDNESDAY   DATE: _____
_____
_____

THURSDAY   DATE: _____
_____
_____

FRIDAY   DATE: _____
_____
_____

SATURDAY   DATE: _____
_____
_____

SUNDAY   DATE: _____
_____
_____

JOURNAL ENTRY

RECALL A TIME WHEN YOU FELT ABSOLUTE JOY; WHAT MADE THAT MOMENT/DAY/TIME JOYOUS?

Monthly BUDGET PLANNER

📅 MONTH (CIRCLE)

JAN	FEB	MAR	APR	MAY	JUN	JUL	AUG	SEP	OCT	NOV	DEC

≔ INCOME

DATE	DESCRIPTION	AMOUNT
	TOTAL:	

🛍 EXPENSES

DATE	DESCRIPTION	AMOUNT
	TOTAL:	

⭐ SUMMARY

TOTAL INCOME	TOTAL EXPENSES	TOTAL SAVINGS

✏ NOTES

_____

_____

_____

_____

_____

YOU CAN REINVENT YOURSELF AS MANY TIMES AS YOU NEED

LEO

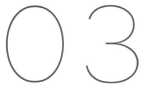

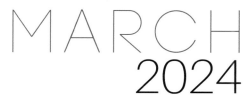

SUNDAY	MONDAY	TUESDAY	WEDNESDAY	THURSDAY	FRIDAY	SATURDAY
					1	2
3	4	5	6	7	8	9
10	11	12	13	14	15	16
17	18	19	20	21	22	23
24	25	26	27	28	29	30
31						

HABITS TO START

- _____
- _____
- _____

SELF-CARE ACTIVITIES

- _____
- _____
- _____

HABITS TO STOP

- _____
- _____
- _____

DON'T FORGET

WEEKLY PLAN

THIS WEEKS PRIORITIES/GOALS

○ _____
○ _____
○ _____
○ _____
○ _____
○ _____
○ _____
○ _____

APPOINTMENTS

○ _____
○ _____
○ _____

REMINDERS

○ _____
○ _____
○ _____

THIS WEEKS
AFFIRMATION/MOTIVATION
_____

_____

_____

MONDAY   DATE: _____
_____
_____

TUESDAY   DATE: _____
_____
_____

WEDNESDAY   DATE: _____
_____
_____

THURSDAY   DATE: _____
_____
_____

FRIDAY   DATE: _____
_____
_____

SATURDAY   DATE: _____
_____
_____

SUNDAY   DATE: _____
_____
_____

WEEKLY PLAN

THIS WEEKS PRIORITIES/GOALS

○ _____
○ _____
○ _____
○ _____
○ _____
○ _____
○ _____
○ _____

APPOINTMENTS

○ _____
○ _____
○ _____

REMINDERS

○ _____
○ _____
○ _____

THIS WEEKS
AFFIRMATION/MOTIVATION
_____

_____

_____

MONDAY   DATE: _____

_____

_____

TUESDAY   DATE: _____

_____

_____

WEDNESDAY   DATE: _____

_____

_____

THURSDAY   DATE: _____

_____

_____

FRIDAY   DATE: _____

_____

_____

SATURDAY   DATE: _____

_____

_____

SUNDAY   DATE: _____

_____

_____

WEEKLY PLAN

THIS WEEKS PRIORITIES/GOALS

○ _____
○ _____
○ _____
○ _____
○ _____
○ _____
○ _____
○ _____

APPOINTMENTS

○ _____
○ _____
○ _____

REMINDERS

○ _____
○ _____
○ _____

THIS WEEKS
AFFIRMATION/MOTIVATION

_____

_____

_____

MONDAY   DATE: _____

_____

_____

TUESDAY   DATE: _____

_____

_____

WEDNESDAY   DATE: _____

_____

_____

THURSDAY   DATE: _____

_____

_____

FRIDAY   DATE: _____

_____

_____

SATURDAY   DATE: _____

_____

_____

SUNDAY   DATE: _____

_____

WEEKLY PLAN

THIS WEEKS PRIORITIES/GOALS

○ _____
○ _____
○ _____
○ _____
○ _____
○ _____
○ _____
○ _____

APPOINTMENTS

○ _____
○ _____
○ _____

REMINDERS

○ _____
○ _____
○ _____

THIS WEEKS
AFFIRMATION/MOTIVATION

_____

_____

_____

_____

MONDAY   DATE: _____

_____

_____

TUESDAY   DATE: _____

_____

_____

WEDNESDAY   DATE: _____

_____

_____

THURSDAY   DATE: _____

_____

_____

FRIDAY   DATE: _____

_____

_____

SATURDAY   DATE: _____

_____

_____

SUNDAY   DATE: _____

_____

_____

JOURNAL ENTRY

IDENTIFY A CURRENT OBSTACLE AND DESCRIBE TWO REALISTIC SOLUTIONS

Monthly BUDGET PLANNER

📅 MONTH (CIRCLE)

JAN	FEB	MAR	APR	MAY	JUN	JUL	AUG	SEP	OCT	NOV	DEC

🗒 INCOME

DATE	DESCRIPTION	AMOUNT
	TOTAL:	

🛍 EXPENSES

DATE	DESCRIPTION	AMOUNT
	TOTAL:	

⭐ SUMMARY

TOTAL INCOME	TOTAL EXPENSES	TOTAL SAVINGS

✏ NOTES

_____

_____

_____

_____

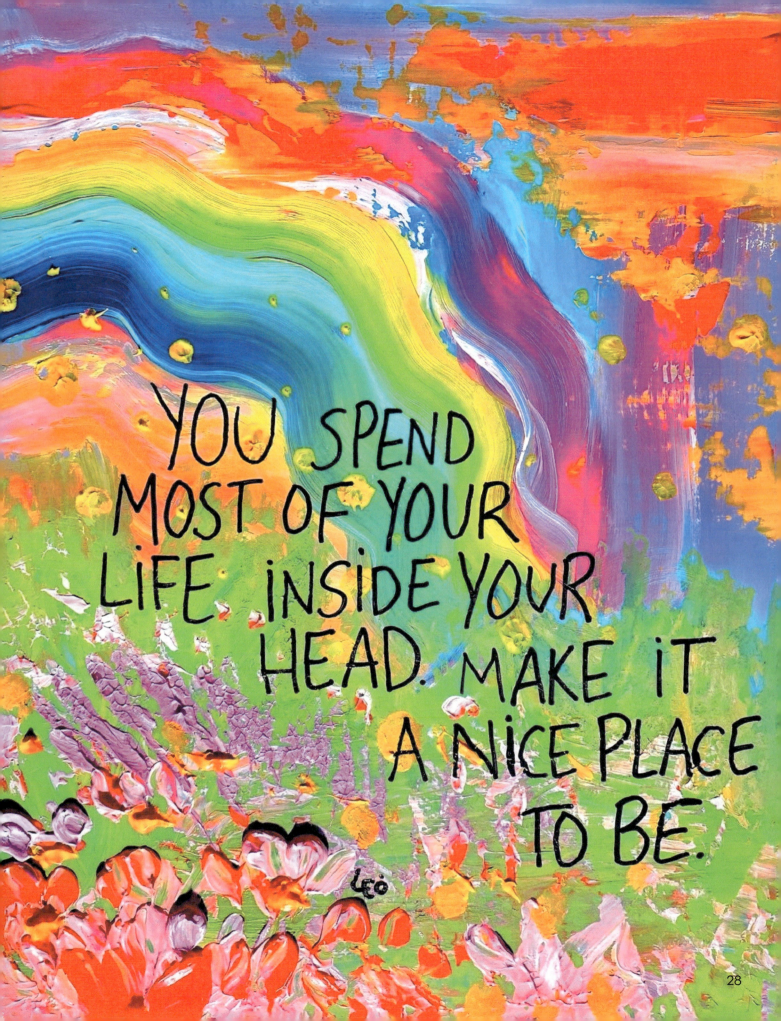

YOU SPEND MOST OF YOUR LIFE INSIDE YOUR HEAD. MAKE IT A NICE PLACE TO BE.

Leo

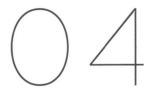 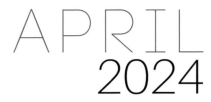

SUNDAY	MONDAY	TUESDAY	WEDNESDAY	THURSDAY	FRIDAY	SATURDAY
	1	2	3	4	5	6
7	8	9	10	11	12	13
14	15	16	17	18	19	20
21	22	23	24	25	26	27
28	29	30				

HABITS TO START

- _____
- _____
- _____

HABITS TO STOP

- _____
- _____
- _____

SELF-CARE ACTIVITIES

- _____
- _____
- _____

DON'T FORGET

WEEKLY PLAN

THIS WEEKS PRIORITIES/GOALS

- ○ _____
- ○ _____
- ○ _____
- ○ _____
- ○ _____
- ○ _____
- ○ _____
- ○ _____

APPOINTMENTS

- ○ _____
- ○ _____
- ○ _____

REMINDERS

- ○ _____
- ○ _____
- ○ _____

THIS WEEKS
AFFIRMATION/MOTIVATION
_____

_____

_____

_____

MONDAY   DATE: _____
_____
_____

TUESDAY   DATE: _____
_____
_____

WEDNESDAY   DATE: _____
_____
_____

THURSDAY   DATE: _____
_____
_____

FRIDAY   DATE: _____
_____
_____

SATURDAY   DATE: _____
_____
_____

SUNDAY   DATE: _____
_____

WEEKLY PLAN

THIS WEEKS PRIORITIES/GOALS

- ◯ _____
- ◯ _____
- ◯ _____
- ◯ _____
- ◯ _____
- ◯ _____
- ◯ _____
- ◯ _____

APPOINTMENTS

- ◯ _____
- ◯ _____
- ◯ _____

REMINDERS

- ◯ _____
- ◯ _____
- ◯ _____

THIS WEEKS
AFFIRMATION/MOTIVATION

_____

_____

_____

MONDAY   DATE: _____

_____

_____

TUESDAY   DATE: _____

_____

_____

WEDNESDAY   DATE: _____

_____

_____

THURSDAY   DATE: _____

_____

_____

FRIDAY   DATE: _____

_____

_____

SATURDAY   DATE: _____

_____

_____

SUNDAY   DATE: _____

_____

_____

WEEKLY PLAN

THIS WEEKS PRIORITIES/GOALS

◯ _____

◯ _____

◯ _____

◯ _____

◯ _____

◯ _____

◯ _____

◯ _____

APPOINTMENTS

◯ _____

◯ _____

◯ _____

REMINDERS

◯ _____

◯ _____

◯ _____

THIS WEEKS
AFFIRMATION/MOTIVATION

_____

_____

_____

MONDAY   DATE: _____

_____

_____

TUESDAY   DATE: _____

_____

_____

WEDNESDAY   DATE: _____

_____

_____

THURSDAY   DATE: _____

_____

_____

FRIDAY   DATE: _____

_____

_____

SATURDAY   DATE: _____

_____

_____

SUNDAY   DATE: _____

_____

_____

WEEKLY PLAN

THIS WEEKS PRIORITIES/GOALS

○ _____
○ _____
○ _____
○ _____
○ _____
○ _____
○ _____
○ _____

APPOINTMENTS

○ _____
○ _____
○ _____

REMINDERS

○ _____
○ _____
○ _____

THIS WEEKS AFFIRMATION/MOTIVATION

_____
_____
_____

MONDAY   DATE: _____

_____
_____

TUESDAY   DATE: _____

_____
_____

WEDNESDAY   DATE: _____

_____
_____

THURSDAY   DATE: _____

_____
_____

FRIDAY   DATE: _____

_____
_____

SATURDAY   DATE: _____

_____
_____

SUNDAY   DATE: _____

_____

WEEKLY PLAN

THIS WEEKS PRIORITIES/GOALS

○ _____
○ _____
○ _____
○ _____
○ _____
○ _____
○ _____
○ _____

APPOINTMENTS

○ _____
○ _____
○ _____

REMINDERS

○ _____
○ _____
○ _____

THIS WEEKS
AFFIRMATION/MOTIVATION

_____

_____

_____

MONDAY   DATE: _____

_____

_____

TUESDAY   DATE: _____

_____

_____

WEDNESDAY   DATE: _____

_____

_____

THURSDAY   DATE: _____

_____

_____

FRIDAY   DATE: _____

_____

_____

SATURDAY   DATE: _____

_____

_____

SUNDAY   DATE: _____

_____

_____

JOURNAL ENTRY

CREATE A SAFE PLACE IN YOUR MIND WITH ONLY YOU. WHAT DO YOU SEE, HEAR, SMELL, FEEL, AND TASTE?

Monthly BUDGET PLANNER

📅 MONTH (CIRCLE)

JAN	FEB	MAR	APR	MAY	JUN	JUL	AUG	SEP	OCT	NOV	DEC

☰ INCOME

DATE	DESCRIPTION	AMOUNT
	TOTAL:	

🛍 EXPENSES

DATE	DESCRIPTION	AMOUNT
	TOTAL:	

⭐ SUMMARY

TOTAL INCOME	TOTAL EXPENSES	TOTAL SAVINGS

✏ NOTES

_____

_____

_____

_____

_____

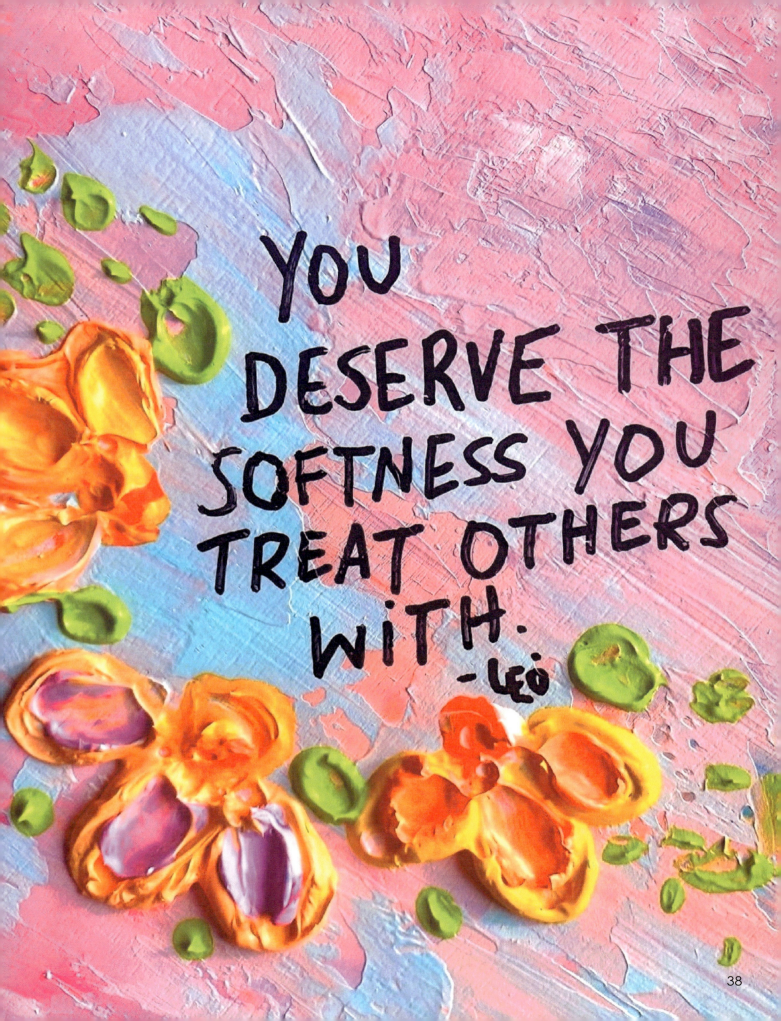

You deserve the softness you treat others with.
— Leo

38

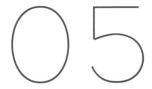

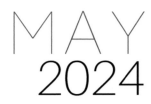

MAY
2024

SUNDAY	MONDAY	TUESDAY	WEDNESDAY	THURSDAY	FRIDAY	SATURDAY
			1	2	3	4
5	6	7	8	9	10	11
12	13	14	15	16	17	18
19	20	21	22	23	24	25
26	27	28	29	30	31	

HABITS TO START

- _____
- _____
- _____

SELF-CARE ACTIVITIES

- _____
- _____
- _____

HABITS TO STOP

- _____
- _____
- _____

DON'T FORGET

WEEKLY PLAN

THIS WEEKS PRIORITIES/GOALS

○ _____
○ _____
○ _____
○ _____
○ _____
○ _____
○ _____
○ _____

APPOINTMENTS

○ _____
○ _____
○ _____

REMINDERS

○ _____
○ _____
○ _____

THIS WEEKS
AFFIRMATION/MOTIVATION

_____

_____

_____

MONDAY   DATE: _____

_____

_____

TUESDAY   DATE: _____

_____

_____

WEDNESDAY   DATE: _____

_____

_____

THURSDAY   DATE: _____

_____

_____

FRIDAY   DATE: _____

_____

_____

SATURDAY   DATE: _____

_____

_____

SUNDAY   DATE: _____

_____

WEEKLY PLAN

THIS WEEKS PRIORITIES/GOALS

○ _____
○ _____
○ _____
○ _____
○ _____
○ _____
○ _____
○ _____

APPOINTMENTS

○ _____
○ _____
○ _____

REMINDERS

○ _____
○ _____
○ _____

THIS WEEKS
AFFIRMATION/MOTIVATION
_____

_____
_____
_____

MONDAY   DATE: _____
_____
_____

TUESDAY   DATE: _____
_____
_____

WEDNESDAY   DATE: _____
_____
_____

THURSDAY   DATE: _____
_____
_____

FRIDAY   DATE: _____
_____
_____

SATURDAY   DATE: _____
_____
_____

SUNDAY   DATE: _____
_____

WEEKLY PLAN

THIS WEEKS PRIORITIES/GOALS

○ _____
○ _____
○ _____
○ _____
○ _____
○ _____
○ _____
○ _____

APPOINTMENTS

○ _____
○ _____
○ _____

REMINDERS

○ _____
○ _____
○ _____

THIS WEEKS
AFFIRMATION/MOTIVATION

_____

_____

_____

MONDAY   DATE: _____

_____

_____

TUESDAY   DATE: _____

_____

_____

WEDNESDAY   DATE: _____

_____

_____

THURSDAY   DATE: _____

_____

_____

FRIDAY   DATE: _____

_____

_____

SATURDAY   DATE: _____

_____

_____

SUNDAY   DATE: _____

_____

WEEKLY PLAN

THIS WEEKS PRIORITIES/GOALS

- _____
- _____
- _____
- _____
- _____
- _____
- _____
- _____

APPOINTMENTS

- _____
- _____
- _____

REMINDERS

- _____
- _____
- _____

THIS WEEKS
AFFIRMATION/MOTIVATION
_____

_____

_____

_____

MONDAY   DATE: _____

_____

_____

TUESDAY   DATE: _____

_____

_____

WEDNESDAY   DATE: _____

_____

_____

THURSDAY   DATE: _____

_____

_____

FRIDAY   DATE: _____

_____

_____

SATURDAY   DATE: _____

_____

_____

SUNDAY   DATE: _____

_____

_____

JOURNAL ENTRY

HOW DO YOU RESPOND WHEN YOU ARE SAD OR FRUSTRATED? IDENTIFY 2 SHORT AND LONG-TERM RESULTS OF THOSE RESPONSES

Monthly BUDGET PLANNER

📅 MONTH (CIRCLE)

JAN	FEB	MAR	APR	MAY	JUN	JUL	AUG	SEP	OCT	NOV	DEC

☰ INCOME

DATE	DESCRIPTION	AMOUNT
	TOTAL:	

🛍 EXPENSES

DATE	DESCRIPTION	AMOUNT
	TOTAL:	

⭐ SUMMARY

TOTAL INCOME	TOTAL EXPENSES	TOTAL SAVINGS

✏ NOTES

_____

_____

_____

_____

_____

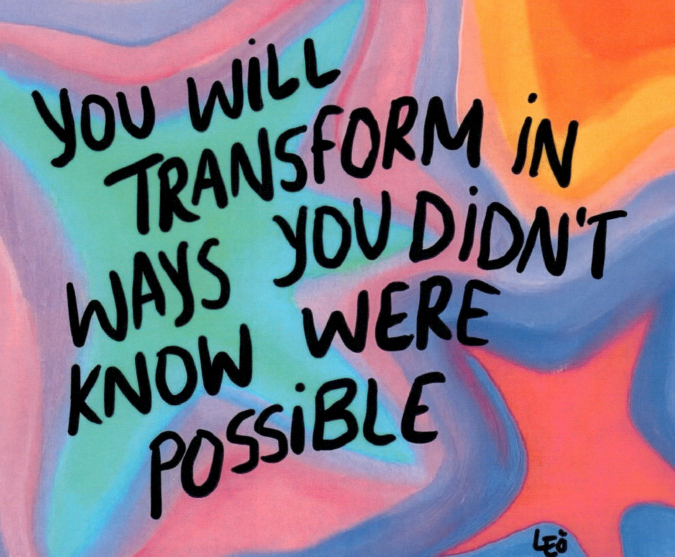

YOU WILL TRANSFORM IN WAYS YOU DIDN'T KNOW WERE POSSIBLE

LEO

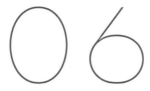

JUNE
2024

SUNDAY	MONDAY	TUESDAY	WEDNESDAY	THURSDAY	FRIDAY	SATURDAY
						1
2	3	4	5	6	7	8
9	10	11	12	13	14	15
16	17	18	19	20	21	22
23 / 30	24	25	26	27	28	29

HABITS TO START

- _____
- _____
- _____

HABITS TO STOP

- _____
- _____
- _____

SELF-CARE ACTIVITIES

- _____
- _____
- _____

DON'T FORGET

WEEKLY PLAN

THIS WEEKS PRIORITIES/GOALS

○ _____
○ _____
○ _____
○ _____
○ _____
○ _____
○ _____
○ _____

APPOINTMENTS

○ _____
○ _____
○ _____

REMINDERS

○ _____
○ _____
○ _____

THIS WEEKS
AFFIRMATION/MOTIVATION

_____

_____

_____

MONDAY   DATE: _____

_____

_____

TUESDAY   DATE: _____

_____

_____

WEDNESDAY   DATE: _____

_____

_____

THURSDAY   DATE: _____

_____

_____

FRIDAY   DATE: _____

_____

_____

SATURDAY   DATE: _____

_____

_____

SUNDAY   DATE: _____

_____

_____

WEEKLY PLAN

THIS WEEKS PRIORITIES/GOALS

○ _____
○ _____
○ _____
○ _____
○ _____
○ _____
○ _____
○ _____

APPOINTMENTS

○ _____
○ _____
○ _____

REMINDERS

○ _____
○ _____
○ _____

THIS WEEKS
AFFIRMATION/MOTIVATION
_____

_____

_____

_____

MONDAY   DATE: _____
_____
_____

TUESDAY   DATE: _____
_____
_____

WEDNESDAY   DATE: _____
_____
_____

THURSDAY   DATE: _____
_____
_____

FRIDAY   DATE: _____
_____
_____

SATURDAY   DATE: _____
_____
_____

SUNDAY   DATE: _____
_____
_____

WEEKLY PLAN

THIS WEEKS PRIORITIES/GOALS

◯ _____

◯ _____

◯ _____

◯ _____

◯ _____

◯ _____

◯ _____

◯ _____

APPOINTMENTS

◯ _____

◯ _____

◯ _____

REMINDERS

◯ _____

◯ _____

◯ _____

THIS WEEKS
AFFIRMATION/MOTIVATION

_____

_____

_____

MONDAY   DATE: _____

_____

_____

TUESDAY   DATE: _____

_____

_____

WEDNESDAY   DATE: _____

_____

_____

THURSDAY   DATE: _____

_____

_____

FRIDAY   DATE: _____

_____

_____

SATURDAY   DATE: _____

_____

_____

SUNDAY   DATE: _____

_____

_____

WEEKLY PLAN

THIS WEEKS PRIORITIES/GOALS

○ _____
○ _____
○ _____
○ _____
○ _____
○ _____
○ _____
○ _____
○ _____

APPOINTMENTS

○ _____
○ _____
○ _____

REMINDERS

○ _____
○ _____
○ _____

THIS WEEKS
AFFIRMATION/MOTIVATION

_____

_____

_____

MONDAY   DATE: _____

_____

_____

TUESDAY   DATE: _____

_____

_____

WEDNESDAY   DATE: _____

_____

_____

THURSDAY   DATE: _____

_____

_____

FRIDAY   DATE: _____

_____

_____

SATURDAY   DATE: _____

_____

_____

SUNDAY   DATE: _____

_____

_____

JOURNAL ENTRY

IDENTIFY 10 (PEOPLE, PLACES, AND/OR THINGS) THAT PROVIDE YOU PEACE AND CALMNESS

Monthly BUDGET PLANNER

📅 MONTH (CIRCLE)

| JAN | FEB | MAR | APR | MAY | JUN | JUL | AUG | SEP | OCT | NOV | DEC |

📋 INCOME

DATE	DESCRIPTION	AMOUNT
	TOTAL:	

🛍️ EXPENSES

DATE	DESCRIPTION	AMOUNT
	TOTAL:	

⭐ SUMMARY

TOTAL INCOME	TOTAL EXPENSES	TOTAL SAVINGS

✏️ NOTES

_____
_____
_____
_____

55

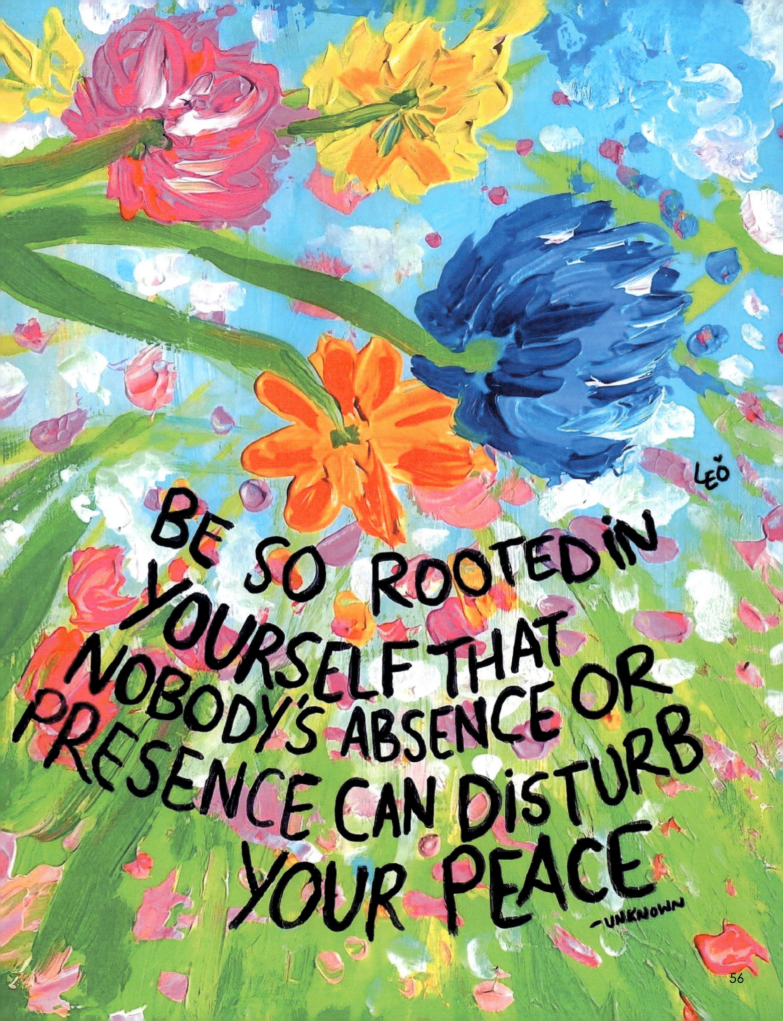

BE SO ROOTED IN YOURSELF THAT NOBODY'S ABSENCE OR PRESENCE CAN DISTURB YOUR PEACE

-UNKNOWN

56

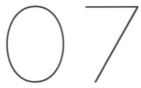

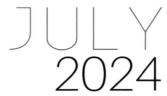

SUNDAY	MONDAY	TUESDAY	WEDNESDAY	THURSDAY	FRIDAY	SATURDAY
	1	2	3	4	5	6
7	8	9	10	11	12	13
14	15	16	17	18	19	20
21	22	23	24	25	26	27
28	29	30	31			

HABITS TO START

- _____
- _____
- _____

HABITS TO STOP

- _____
- _____
- _____

SELF-CARE ACTIVITIES

- _____
- _____
- _____

DON'T FORGET

WEEKLY PLAN

THIS WEEKS PRIORITIES/GOALS

- _____
- _____
- _____
- _____
- _____
- _____
- _____
- _____

APPOINTMENTS

- _____
- _____
- _____

REMINDERS

- _____
- _____
- _____

THIS WEEKS
AFFIRMATION/MOTIVATION

_____

_____

_____

_____

MONDAY   DATE: _____

_____

_____

TUESDAY   DATE: _____

_____

_____

WEDNESDAY   DATE: _____

_____

_____

THURSDAY   DATE: _____

_____

_____

FRIDAY   DATE: _____

_____

_____

SATURDAY   DATE: _____

_____

_____

SUNDAY   DATE: _____

_____

_____

WEEKLY PLAN

THIS WEEKS PRIORITIES/GOALS

○ _____
○ _____
○ _____
○ _____
○ _____
○ _____
○ _____
○ _____

APPOINTMENTS

○ _____
○ _____
○ _____

REMINDERS

○ _____
○ _____
○ _____

THIS WEEKS
AFFIRMATION/MOTIVATION
_____
_____
_____

MONDAY   DATE: _____
_____
_____

TUESDAY   DATE: _____
_____
_____

WEDNESDAY   DATE: _____
_____
_____

THURSDAY   DATE: _____
_____
_____

FRIDAY   DATE: _____
_____
_____

SATURDAY   DATE: _____
_____
_____

SUNDAY   DATE: _____
_____
_____

WEEKLY PLAN

THIS WEEKS PRIORITIES/GOALS

○ _____

○ _____

○ _____

○ _____

○ _____

○ _____

○ _____

○ _____

APPOINTMENTS

○ _____

○ _____

○ _____

REMINDERS

○ _____

○ _____

○ _____

THIS WEEKS
AFFIRMATION/MOTIVATION
_____

_____

_____

_____

MONDAY   DATE: _____

_____

_____

TUESDAY   DATE: _____

_____

_____

WEDNESDAY   DATE: _____

_____

_____

THURSDAY   DATE: _____

_____

_____

FRIDAY   DATE: _____

_____

_____

SATURDAY   DATE: _____

_____

_____

SUNDAY   DATE: _____

_____

_____

WEEKLY PLAN

THIS WEEKS PRIORITIES/GOALS

◯ _____
◯ _____
◯ _____
◯ _____
◯ _____
◯ _____
◯ _____
◯ _____

APPOINTMENTS

◯ _____
◯ _____
◯ _____

REMINDERS

◯ _____
◯ _____
◯ _____

THIS WEEKS
AFFIRMATION/MOTIVATION

_____

_____

_____

MONDAY   DATE: _____

_____

_____

TUESDAY   DATE: _____

_____

_____

WEDNESDAY   DATE: _____

_____

_____

THURSDAY   DATE: _____

_____

_____

FRIDAY   DATE: _____

_____

_____

SATURDAY   DATE: _____

_____

_____

SUNDAY   DATE: _____

_____

_____

WEEKLY PLAN

THIS WEEKS PRIORITIES/GOALS

○ _____
○ _____
○ _____
○ _____
○ _____
○ _____
○ _____
○ _____

APPOINTMENTS

○ _____
○ _____
○ _____

REMINDERS

○ _____
○ _____
○ _____

THIS WEEKS
AFFIRMATION/MOTIVATION

_____

_____

_____

MONDAY   DATE: _____

_____

_____

TUESDAY   DATE: _____

_____

_____

WEDNESDAY   DATE: _____

_____

_____

THURSDAY   DATE: _____

_____

_____

FRIDAY   DATE: _____

_____

_____

SATURDAY   DATE: _____

_____

_____

SUNDAY   DATE: _____

_____

JOURNAL ENTRY (FILL IN THE BLANK)

THIS MONTH I CHOSE TO PRACTICE THE VALUE OF _ _ _ _ _ _ _ _ _ _ _ _ _ _ _ BECAUSE:

Monthly BUDGET PLANNER

📅 **MONTH (CIRCLE)**

JAN	FEB	MAR	APR	MAY	JUN	JUL	AUG	SEP	OCT	NOV	DEC

☰ **INCOME**

DATE	DESCRIPTION	AMOUNT
	TOTAL:	

🛍 **EXPENSES**

DATE	DESCRIPTION	AMOUNT
	TOTAL:	

⭐ **SUMMARY**

TOTAL INCOME	TOTAL EXPENSES	TOTAL SAVINGS

✏ **NOTES**

_____

_____

_____

_____

65

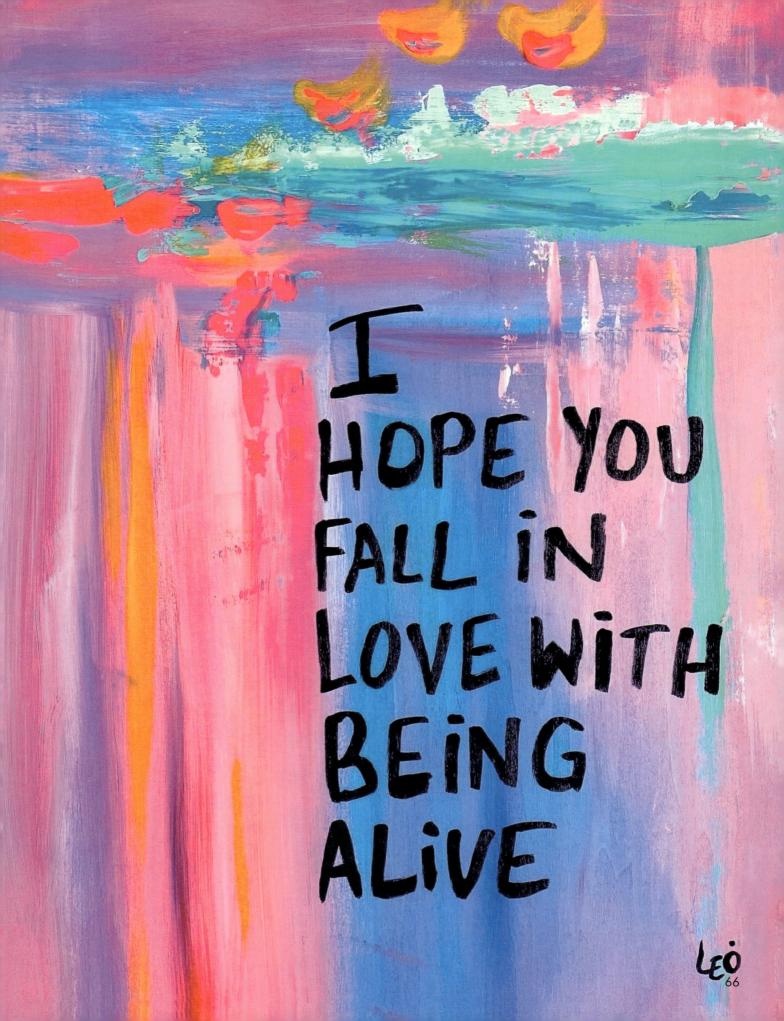

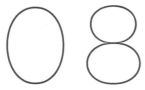

08

AUGUST
2024

SUNDAY	MONDAY	TUESDAY	WEDNESDAY	THURSDAY	FRIDAY	SATURDAY
				1	2	3
4	5	6	7	8	9	10
11	12	13	14	15	16	17
18	19	20	21	22	23	24
25	26	27	28	29	30	31

HABITS TO START

- _____
- _____
- _____

SELF-CARE ACTIVITIES

- _____
- _____
- _____

HABITS TO STOP

- _____
- _____
- _____

DON'T FORGET

WEEKLY PLAN

THIS WEEKS PRIORITIES/GOALS

○ _____
○ _____
○ _____
○ _____
○ _____
○ _____
○ _____
○ _____

APPOINTMENTS

○ _____
○ _____
○ _____

REMINDERS

○ _____
○ _____
○ _____

THIS WEEKS
AFFIRMATION/MOTIVATION
_____

_____
_____
_____

MONDAY   DATE: _____
_____
_____

TUESDAY   DATE: _____
_____
_____

WEDNESDAY   DATE: _____
_____
_____

THURSDAY   DATE: _____
_____
_____

FRIDAY   DATE: _____
_____
_____

SATURDAY   DATE: _____
_____
_____

SUNDAY   DATE: _____
_____

WEEKLY PLAN

THIS WEEKS PRIORITIES/GOALS

○ _____

○ _____

○ _____

○ _____

○ _____

○ _____

○ _____

○ _____

APPOINTMENTS

○ _____

○ _____

○ _____

REMINDERS

○ _____

○ _____

○ _____

THIS WEEKS
AFFIRMATION/MOTIVATION

_____

_____

_____

MONDAY   DATE: _____

_____

_____

TUESDAY   DATE: _____

_____

_____

WEDNESDAY   DATE: _____

_____

_____

THURSDAY   DATE: _____

_____

_____

FRIDAY   DATE: _____

_____

_____

SATURDAY   DATE: _____

_____

_____

SUNDAY   DATE: _____

_____

_____

WEEKLY PLAN

THIS WEEKS PRIORITIES/GOALS

○ _____
○ _____
○ _____
○ _____
○ _____
○ _____
○ _____
○ _____

APPOINTMENTS

○ _____
○ _____
○ _____

REMINDERS

○ _____
○ _____
○ _____

THIS WEEKS
AFFIRMATION/MOTIVATION
_____

_____

_____

_____

MONDAY   DATE: _____
_____
_____

TUESDAY   DATE: _____
_____
_____

WEDNESDAY   DATE: _____
_____
_____

THURSDAY   DATE: _____
_____
_____

FRIDAY   DATE: _____
_____
_____

SATURDAY   DATE: _____
_____
_____

SUNDAY   DATE: _____
_____
_____

WEEKLY PLAN

THIS WEEKS PRIORITIES/GOALS

○ _____
○ _____
○ _____
○ _____
○ _____
○ _____
○ _____
○ _____

APPOINTMENTS

○ _____
○ _____
○ _____

REMINDERS

○ _____
○ _____
○ _____

THIS WEEKS
AFFIRMATION/MOTIVATION
_____

_____

_____

_____

MONDAY   DATE: _____

_____

_____

TUESDAY   DATE: _____

_____

_____

WEDNESDAY   DATE: _____

_____

_____

THURSDAY   DATE: _____

_____

_____

FRIDAY   DATE: _____

_____

_____

SATURDAY   DATE: _____

_____

_____

SUNDAY   DATE: _____

_____

_____

JOURNAL ENTRY

**HOW DOES A LIFE WORTH LIVING LOOK TO YOU?
ARE YOU LIVING THIS LIFE? IF NOT, WHY?**

Monthly BUDGET PLANNER

📅 MONTH (CIRCLE)

| JAN | FEB | MAR | APR | MAY | JUN | JUL | AUG | SEP | OCT | NOV | DEC |

☰ INCOME

DATE	DESCRIPTION	AMOUNT
	TOTAL:	

🛍 EXPENSES

DATE	DESCRIPTION	AMOUNT
	TOTAL:	

⭐ SUMMARY

TOTAL INCOME	TOTAL EXPENSES	TOTAL SAVINGS

✏ NOTES

_____

_____

_____

_____

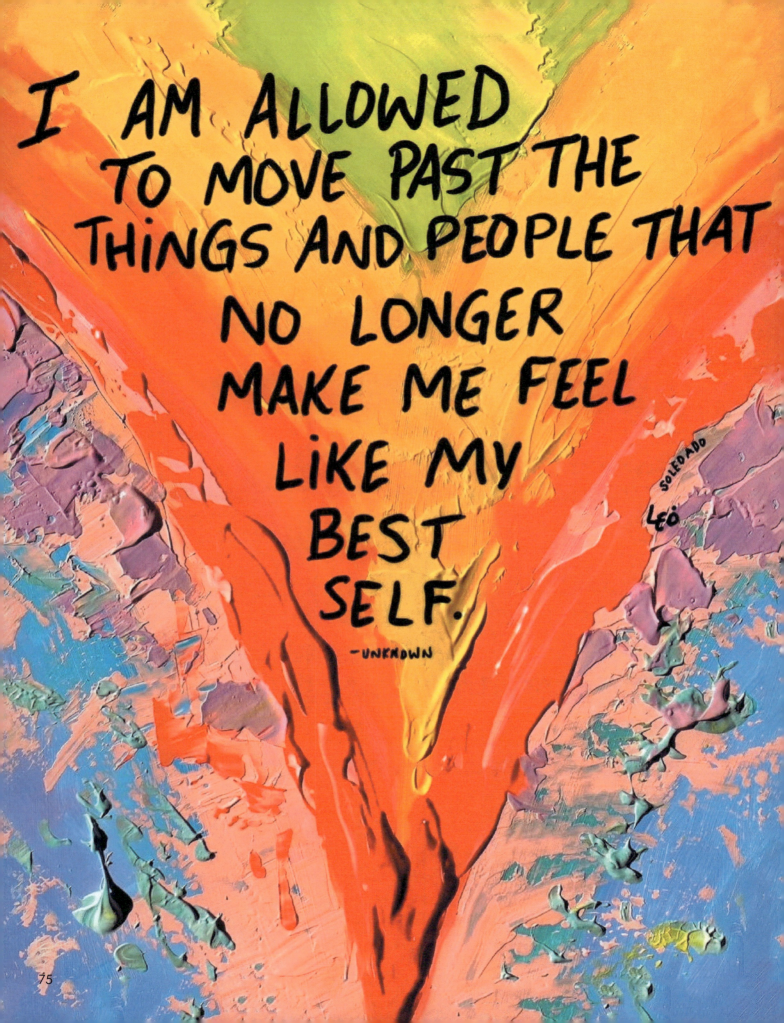

I AM ALLOWED TO MOVE PAST THE THINGS AND PEOPLE THAT NO LONGER MAKE ME FEEL LIKE MY BEST SELF.

—UNKNOWN

SOLEDADO

LEO

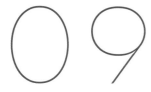

SEPTEMBER
2024

SUNDAY	MONDAY	TUESDAY	WEDNESDAY	THURSDAY	FRIDAY	SATURDAY
1	2	3	4	5	6	7
8	9	10	11	12	13	14
15	16	17	18	19	20	21
22	23	24	25	26	27	28
29	30					

HABITS TO START

- _____
- _____
- _____

SELF-CARE ACTIVITIES

- _____
- _____
- _____

HABITS TO STOP

- _____
- _____
- _____

DON'T FORGET

WEEKLY PLAN

THIS WEEKS PRIORITIES/GOALS

○ _____
○ _____
○ _____
○ _____
○ _____
○ _____
○ _____
○ _____

APPOINTMENTS

○ _____
○ _____
○ _____

REMINDERS

○ _____
○ _____
○ _____

THIS WEEKS
AFFIRMATION/MOTIVATION

_____
_____
_____

MONDAY   DATE: _____

_____
_____

TUESDAY   DATE: _____

_____
_____

WEDNESDAY   DATE: _____

_____
_____

THURSDAY   DATE: _____

_____
_____

FRIDAY   DATE: _____

_____
_____

SATURDAY   DATE: _____

_____
_____

SUNDAY   DATE: _____

_____
_____

WEEKLY PLAN

THIS WEEKS PRIORITIES/GOALS

○ _____

○ _____

○ _____

○ _____

○ _____

○ _____

○ _____

○ _____

APPOINTMENTS

○ _____

○ _____

○ _____

REMINDERS

○ _____

○ _____

○ _____

THIS WEEKS
AFFIRMATION/MOTIVATION
_____

_____

_____

_____

MONDAY   DATE: _____

_____

_____

TUESDAY   DATE: _____

_____

_____

WEDNESDAY   DATE: _____

_____

_____

THURSDAY   DATE: _____

_____

_____

FRIDAY   DATE: _____

_____

_____

SATURDAY   DATE: _____

_____

_____

SUNDAY   DATE: _____

_____

_____

WEEKLY PLAN

THIS WEEKS PRIORITIES/GOALS

○ _____
○ _____
○ _____
○ _____
○ _____
○ _____
○ _____
○ _____

APPOINTMENTS

○ _____
○ _____
○ _____

REMINDERS

○ _____
○ _____
○ _____

THIS WEEKS
AFFIRMATION/MOTIVATION
_____

_____

_____

MONDAY   DATE: _____
_____
_____

TUESDAY   DATE: _____
_____
_____

WEDNESDAY   DATE: _____
_____
_____

THURSDAY   DATE: _____
_____
_____

FRIDAY   DATE: _____
_____
_____

SATURDAY   DATE: _____
_____
_____

SUNDAY   DATE: _____
_____
_____

WEEKLY PLAN

THIS WEEKS PRIORITIES/GOALS

- ⃝ _____
- ⃝ _____
- ⃝ _____
- ⃝ _____
- ⃝ _____
- ⃝ _____
- ⃝ _____
- ⃝ _____

APPOINTMENTS

- ⃝ _____
- ⃝ _____
- ⃝ _____

REMINDERS

- ⃝ _____
- ⃝ _____
- ⃝ _____

THIS WEEKS
AFFIRMATION/MOTIVATION

_____

_____

_____

MONDAY   DATE: _____

_____

_____

TUESDAY   DATE: _____

_____

_____

WEDNESDAY   DATE: _____

_____

_____

THURSDAY   DATE: _____

_____

_____

FRIDAY   DATE: _____

_____

_____

SATURDAY   DATE: _____

_____

_____

SUNDAY   DATE: _____

_____

_____

JOURNAL ENTRY

IDENTIFY A MEANINGFUL PERSON IN YOUR LIFE. HOW DOES THIS PERSON ADD MEANING TO YOUR LIFE?

Monthly BUDGET PLANNER

📅 MONTH (CIRCLE)

JAN	FEB	MAR	APR	MAY	JUN	JUL	AUG	SEP	OCT	NOV	DEC

☰ INCOME

DATE	DESCRIPTION	AMOUNT
	TOTAL:	

🛍 EXPENSES

DATE	DESCRIPTION	AMOUNT
	TOTAL:	

⭐ SUMMARY

TOTAL INCOME	TOTAL EXPENSES	TOTAL SAVINGS

✏ NOTES

_____

_____

_____

_____

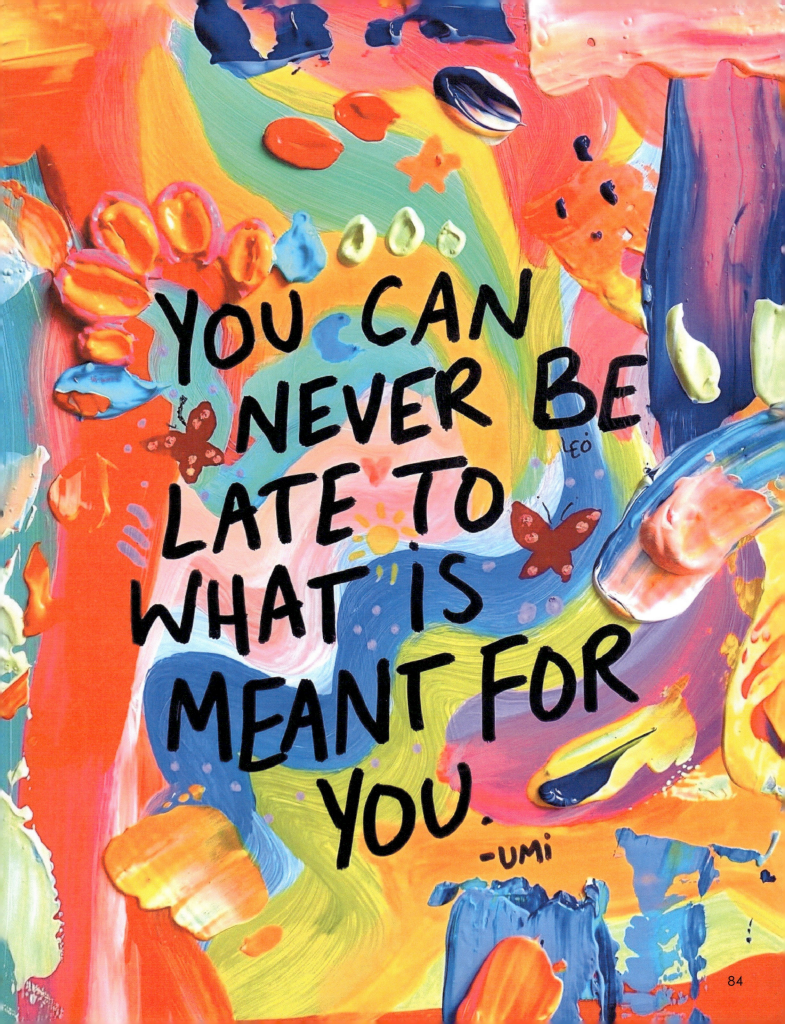

YOU CAN NEVER BE LATE TO WHAT IS MEANT FOR YOU.

-UMI

84

10

OCTOBER
2024

SUNDAY	MONDAY	TUESDAY	WEDNESDAY	THURSDAY	FRIDAY	SATURDAY
		1	2	3	4	5
6	7	8	9	10	11	12
13	14	15	16	17	18	19
20	21	22	23	24	25	26
27	28	29	30	31		

HABITS TO START

- _____
- _____
- _____

HABITS TO STOP

- _____
- _____
- _____

SELF-CARE ACTIVITIES

- _____
- _____
- _____

DON'T FORGET

WEEKLY PLAN

THIS WEEKS PRIORITIES/GOALS

○ _____
○ _____
○ _____
○ _____
○ _____
○ _____
○ _____
○ _____

APPOINTMENTS

○ _____
○ _____
○ _____

REMINDERS

○ _____
○ _____
○ _____

THIS WEEKS
AFFIRMATION/MOTIVATION

_____

_____

_____

MONDAY   DATE: _____

_____

_____

TUESDAY   DATE: _____

_____

_____

WEDNESDAY   DATE: _____

_____

_____

THURSDAY   DATE: _____

_____

_____

FRIDAY   DATE: _____

_____

_____

SATURDAY   DATE: _____

_____

_____

SUNDAY   DATE: _____

_____

_____

WEEKLY PLAN

THIS WEEKS PRIORITIES/GOALS

- ○ _____
- ○ _____
- ○ _____
- ○ _____
- ○ _____
- ○ _____
- ○ _____
- ○ _____

APPOINTMENTS

- ○ _____
- ○ _____
- ○ _____

REMINDERS

- ○ _____
- ○ _____
- ○ _____

THIS WEEKS
AFFIRMATION/MOTIVATION
_____
_____
_____
_____

MONDAY   DATE: _____
_____
_____

TUESDAY   DATE: _____
_____
_____

WEDNESDAY   DATE: _____
_____
_____

THURSDAY   DATE: _____
_____
_____

FRIDAY   DATE: _____
_____
_____

SATURDAY   DATE: _____
_____
_____

SUNDAY   DATE: _____
_____

WEEKLY PLAN

THIS WEEKS PRIORITIES/GOALS

○ _____

○ _____

○ _____

○ _____

○ _____

○ _____

○ _____

○ _____

APPOINTMENTS

○ _____

○ _____

○ _____

REMINDERS

○ _____

○ _____

○ _____

THIS WEEKS
AFFIRMATION/MOTIVATION

_____

_____

_____

MONDAY   DATE: _____

_____

_____

TUESDAY   DATE: _____

_____

_____

WEDNESDAY   DATE: _____

_____

_____

THURSDAY   DATE: _____

_____

_____

FRIDAY   DATE: _____

_____

_____

SATURDAY   DATE: _____

_____

_____

SUNDAY   DATE: _____

_____

_____

WEEKLY PLAN

THIS WEEKS PRIORITIES/GOALS

○ _____

○ _____

○ _____

○ _____

○ _____

○ _____

○ _____

○ _____

APPOINTMENTS

○ _____

○ _____

○ _____

REMINDERS

○ _____

○ _____

○ _____

THIS WEEKS
AFFIRMATION/MOTIVATION

_____

_____

_____

MONDAY   DATE: _____

_____

_____

TUESDAY   DATE: _____

_____

_____

WEDNESDAY   DATE: _____

_____

_____

THURSDAY   DATE: _____

_____

_____

FRIDAY   DATE: _____

_____

_____

SATURDAY   DATE: _____

_____

_____

SUNDAY   DATE: _____

_____

_____

WEEKLY PLAN

THIS WEEKS PRIORITIES/GOALS

○ _____
○ _____
○ _____
○ _____
○ _____
○ _____
○ _____
○ _____

APPOINTMENTS

○ _____
○ _____
○ _____

REMINDERS

○ _____
○ _____
○ _____

THIS WEEKS
AFFIRMATION/MOTIVATION

_____

_____

_____

MONDAY   DATE: _____

_____

_____

TUESDAY   DATE: _____

_____

_____

WEDNESDAY   DATE: _____

_____

_____

THURSDAY   DATE: _____

_____

_____

FRIDAY   DATE: _____

_____

_____

SATURDAY   DATE: _____

_____

_____

SUNDAY   DATE: _____

_____

JOURNAL ENTRY

HOW DO YOU KNOW WHEN YOU ARE STRESSED?
WHAT IS YOUR IDEAL WAY TO RELIEVE STRESS?

Monthly BUDGET PLANNER

📅 MONTH (CIRCLE)

JAN	FEB	MAR	APR	MAY	JUN	JUL	AUG	SEP	OCT	NOV	DEC

☰ INCOME

DATE	DESCRIPTION	AMOUNT
	TOTAL:	

🛍 EXPENSES

DATE	DESCRIPTION	AMOUNT
	TOTAL:	

★ SUMMARY

TOTAL INCOME	TOTAL EXPENSES	TOTAL SAVINGS

✏ NOTES

_____

_____

_____

_____

THE RESULTS OF YOUR HEALING ARE SHOWING

KEEP GOING.

Leo

11

NOVEMBER
2024

SUNDAY	MONDAY	TUESDAY	WEDNESDAY	THURSDAY	FRIDAY	SATURDAY
					1	2
3	4	5	6	7	8	9
10	11	12	13	14	15	16
17	18	19	20	21	22	23
24	25	26	27	28	29	30

HABITS TO START

- _____
- _____
- _____

HABITS TO STOP

- _____
- _____
- _____

SELF-CARE ACTIVITIES

- _____
- _____
- _____

DON'T FORGET

WEEKLY PLAN

THIS WEEKS PRIORITIES/GOALS

○ _____
○ _____
○ _____
○ _____
○ _____
○ _____
○ _____
○ _____

APPOINTMENTS

○ _____
○ _____
○ _____

REMINDERS

○ _____
○ _____
○ _____

THIS WEEKS
AFFIRMATION/MOTIVATION

_____

_____

_____

MONDAY   DATE: _____

_____

_____

TUESDAY   DATE: _____

_____

_____

WEDNESDAY   DATE: _____

_____

_____

THURSDAY   DATE: _____

_____

_____

FRIDAY   DATE: _____

_____

_____

SATURDAY   DATE: _____

_____

_____

SUNDAY   DATE: _____

_____

_____

WEEKLY PLAN

THIS WEEKS PRIORITIES/GOALS

○ _____
○ _____
○ _____
○ _____
○ _____
○ _____
○ _____
○ _____

APPOINTMENTS

○ _____
○ _____
○ _____

REMINDERS

○ _____
○ _____
○ _____

THIS WEEKS
AFFIRMATION/MOTIVATION
_____

_____

_____

MONDAY   DATE: _____
_____
_____

TUESDAY   DATE: _____
_____
_____

WEDNESDAY   DATE: _____
_____
_____

THURSDAY   DATE: _____
_____
_____

FRIDAY   DATE: _____
_____
_____

SATURDAY   DATE: _____
_____
_____

SUNDAY   DATE: _____
_____
_____

WEEKLY PLAN

THIS WEEKS PRIORITIES/GOALS

○ _____
○ _____
○ _____
○ _____
○ _____
○ _____
○ _____
○ _____

APPOINTMENTS

○ _____
○ _____
○ _____

REMINDERS

○ _____
○ _____
○ _____

THIS WEEKS
AFFIRMATION/MOTIVATION

_____

_____

_____

MONDAY   DATE: _____

_____

_____

TUESDAY   DATE: _____

_____

_____

WEDNESDAY   DATE: _____

_____

_____

THURSDAY   DATE: _____

_____

_____

FRIDAY   DATE: _____

_____

_____

SATURDAY   DATE: _____

_____

_____

SUNDAY   DATE: _____

_____

_____

WEEKLY PLAN

THIS WEEKS PRIORITIES/GOALS

○ _____

○ _____

○ _____

○ _____

○ _____

○ _____

○ _____

○ _____

APPOINTMENTS

○ _____

○ _____

○ _____

REMINDERS

○ _____

○ _____

○ _____

THIS WEEKS
AFFIRMATION/MOTIVATION
_____

_____

_____

MONDAY   DATE: _____

_____

_____

TUESDAY   DATE: _____

_____

_____

WEDNESDAY   DATE: _____

_____

_____

THURSDAY   DATE: _____

_____

_____

FRIDAY   DATE: _____

_____

_____

SATURDAY   DATE: _____

_____

_____

SUNDAY   DATE: _____

_____

_____

JOURNAL ENTRY

HOW DO YOU RESPOND TO REJECTION?
HOW DO YOU RESPOND TO CORRECTION/CRITICISM?
IF YOU DESIRE TO CHANGE YOUR RESPONSE, HOW WOULD YOU LIKE IT TO CHANGE?

Monthly BUDGET PLANNER

📅 MONTH (CIRCLE)

JAN	FEB	MAR	APR	MAY	JUN	JUL	AUG	SEP	OCT	NOV	DEC

☰ INCOME

DATE	DESCRIPTION	AMOUNT
	TOTAL:	

🛍 EXPENSES

DATE	DESCRIPTION	AMOUNT
	TOTAL:	

⭐ SUMMARY

TOTAL INCOME	TOTAL EXPENSES	TOTAL SAVINGS

✏ NOTES

_____

_____

_____

_____

_____

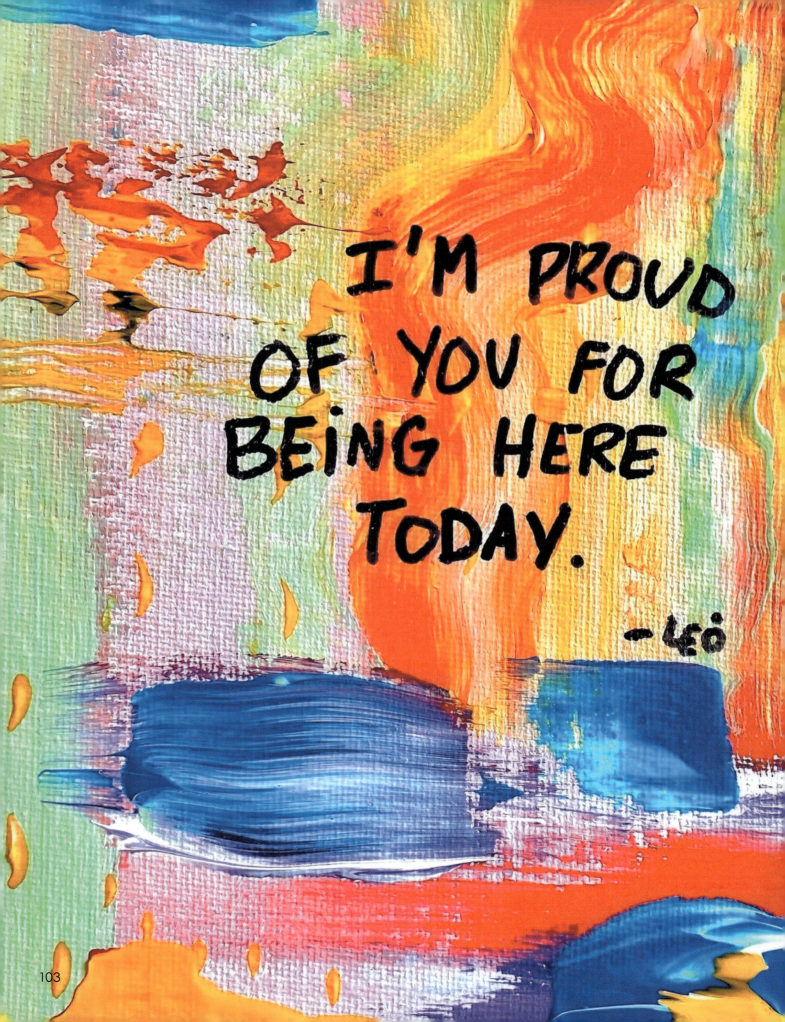

I'M PROUD OF YOU FOR BEING HERE TODAY.

—LEO

103

12 DECEMBER 2024

SUNDAY	MONDAY	TUESDAY	WEDNESDAY	THURSDAY	FRIDAY	SATURDAY
1	2	3	4	5	6	7
8	9	10	11	12	13	14
15	16	17	18	19	20	21
22	23	24	25	26	27	28
29	30	31				

HABITS TO START

- _____
- _____
- _____

HABITS TO STOP

- _____
- _____
- _____

SELF-CARE ACTIVITIES

- _____
- _____
- _____

DON'T FORGET

WEEKLY PLAN

THIS WEEKS PRIORITIES/GOALS

○ _____
○ _____
○ _____
○ _____
○ _____
○ _____
○ _____
○ _____

APPOINTMENTS

○ _____
○ _____
○ _____

REMINDERS

○ _____
○ _____
○ _____

THIS WEEKS
AFFIRMATION/MOTIVATION
_____
_____
_____

MONDAY   DATE: _____
_____
_____

TUESDAY   DATE: _____
_____
_____

WEDNESDAY   DATE: _____
_____
_____

THURSDAY   DATE: _____
_____
_____

FRIDAY   DATE: _____
_____
_____

SATURDAY   DATE: _____
_____
_____

SUNDAY   DATE: _____
_____

WEEKLY PLAN

THIS WEEKS PRIORITIES/GOALS

○ _____
○ _____
○ _____
○ _____
○ _____
○ _____
○ _____
○ _____

APPOINTMENTS

○ _____
○ _____
○ _____

REMINDERS

○ _____
○ _____
○ _____

THIS WEEKS
AFFIRMATION/MOTIVATION

_____

_____

_____

MONDAY   DATE: _____

_____

_____

TUESDAY   DATE: _____

_____

_____

WEDNESDAY   DATE: _____

_____

_____

THURSDAY   DATE: _____

_____

_____

FRIDAY   DATE: _____

_____

_____

SATURDAY   DATE: _____

_____

_____

SUNDAY   DATE: _____

_____

_____

WEEKLY PLAN

THIS WEEKS PRIORITIES/GOALS

○ _____
○ _____
○ _____
○ _____
○ _____
○ _____
○ _____
○ _____

APPOINTMENTS

○ _____
○ _____
○ _____

REMINDERS

○ _____
○ _____
○ _____

THIS WEEKS
AFFIRMATION/MOTIVATION

_____

_____

_____

MONDAY   DATE: _____

_____

_____

TUESDAY   DATE: _____

_____

_____

WEDNESDAY   DATE: _____

_____

_____

THURSDAY   DATE: _____

_____

_____

FRIDAY   DATE: _____

_____

_____

SATURDAY   DATE: _____

_____

_____

SUNDAY   DATE: _____

_____

_____

WEEKLY PLAN

THIS WEEKS PRIORITIES/GOALS

◯ _____
◯ _____
◯ _____
◯ _____
◯ _____
◯ _____
◯ _____
◯ _____

APPOINTMENTS

◯ _____
◯ _____
◯ _____

REMINDERS

◯ _____
◯ _____
◯ _____

THIS WEEKS
AFFIRMATION/MOTIVATION
_____

_____

_____

_____

MONDAY   DATE: _____
_____
_____

TUESDAY   DATE: _____
_____
_____

WEDNESDAY   DATE: _____
_____
_____

THURSDAY   DATE: _____
_____
_____

FRIDAY   DATE: _____
_____
_____

SATURDAY   DATE: _____
_____
_____

SUNDAY   DATE: _____
_____
_____

WEEKLY PLAN

THIS WEEKS PRIORITIES/GOALS

- ○ _____
- ○ _____
- ○ _____
- ○ _____
- ○ _____
- ○ _____
- ○ _____
- ○ _____

APPOINTMENTS

- ○ _____
- ○ _____
- ○ _____

REMINDERS

- ○ _____
- ○ _____
- ○ _____

THIS WEEKS
AFFIRMATION/MOTIVATION

_____

_____

_____

MONDAY   DATE: _____

_____

_____

TUESDAY   DATE: _____

_____

_____

WEDNESDAY   DATE: _____

_____

_____

THURSDAY   DATE: _____

_____

_____

FRIDAY   DATE: _____

_____

_____

SATURDAY   DATE: _____

_____

_____

SUNDAY   DATE: _____

_____

_____

JOURNAL ENTRY

WHAT ARE 3 THINGS YOU ARE MOST PROUD OF, AND WHY?

Monthly BUDGET PLANNER

📅 MONTH (CIRCLE)

JAN	FEB	MAR	APR	MAY	JUN	JUL	AUG	SEP	OCT	NOV	DEC

≔ INCOME

DATE	DESCRIPTION	AMOUNT
	TOTAL:	

🛍 EXPENSES

DATE	DESCRIPTION	AMOUNT
	TOTAL:	

★ SUMMARY

TOTAL INCOME	TOTAL EXPENSES	TOTAL SAVINGS

✏ NOTES

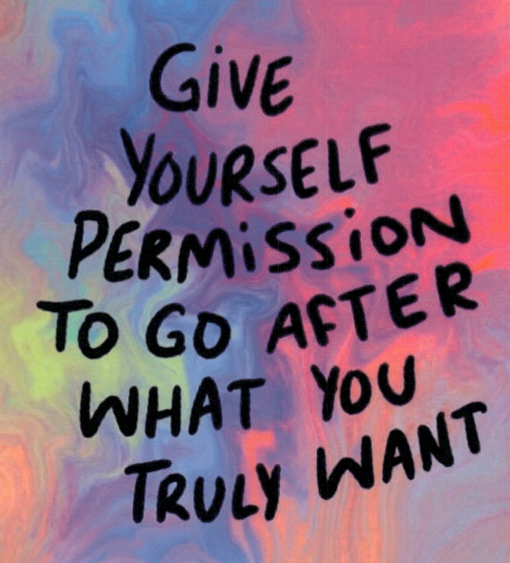

GIVE YOURSELF PERMISSION TO GO AFTER WHAT YOU TRULY WANT

LEO

○ ....

○ ....

○ ....

○ ....

○ ....

○ ....

○ ....

○ ....

○ ....

○ ....

○ ....

○ ....

○ ....

○ ....

○ ....

○ ....

○ ....

○ ....

○ ....

○ ....

○ ....

ABOUT the AUTHOR

Jasmin is the CEO and Owner of Elevated Wellness Counseling & Consulting. She is a Licensed Professional Counselor and Licensed Chemical Dependency Counselor in the state of Texas. Jasmin specializes in Depression, Anxiety, Trauma, Mood Disorders, and Chemical Dependency.

Throughout her life, she's confronted depression, anxiety, suicidal thoughts, and sexual trauma. These experiences were challenging but Jasmin developed a healthy way to use her lessons in life to help others navigate their life. She became a counselor to create safe spaces for others to be heard, healed, and rediscover hope in their lives.

In life, we wear many hats and it's difficult to gain control when the past, present, and future are all competing for attention. Jasmin is a mother, daughter, friend, sister, businesswoman, therapist, mentor, etc., and as many know, the chaos of the hats can be overwhelming. Therefore, utilizing planners, agendas, organizers, and journals became her norm. Jasmin discovered that weekly planning was the most effective for productivity. Journaling is a mindfulness tool Jasmin's used since childhood to help organize her thoughts and emotions. Calendars have a beneficial layout for planning and organizing.

Combining the organizational structure of a planner and the cathartic release of the journal was transformational.

In spite of your life journey, know and believe it is not over, for it is just the beginning. You have the power and now a tool to conquer all your heart desires. Let go of any shame or guilt that you may feel and thank yourself for taking a monumental step towards wellness. You can and will do great things! You Got This!

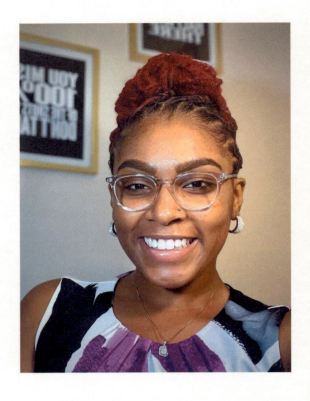

FEEL FREE TO FOLLOW ME ON SOCIAL MEDIA:

INSTAGRAM-
@ELEVATEDWELLNESS365
@JASTHETHERAPIST

FACEBOOK-
ELEVATED WELLNESS
COUNSELING & CONSULTING

WEBSITE-
WWW.ELEVATEDWELLNESS365.COM

Archway Publishing books may be ordered through booksellers or by contacting:

Archway Publishing
1663 Liberty Drive
Bloomington, IN 47403
www.archwaypublishing.com
844-669-3957

ISBN: 978-1-6657-5812-3 (sc)
ISBN: 978-1-6657-5813-0 (e)

Library of Congress Control Number: 2024905191

Print information available on the last page.

Archway Publishing rev. date: 04/09/2024

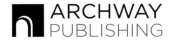

Printed in the United States
by Baker & Taylor Publisher Services